Zied Hadrich
Maissa Bellaaj

BLEEDING AFTER CEPHALIC DUODENO-PANCREATECTOMY

Zied Hadrich
Maissa Bellaaj

BLEEDING AFTER CEPHALIC DUODENO-PANCREATECTOMY

INCIDENCE, RISK FACTORS AND PROGNOSTIC IMPACT

ScienciaScripts

Imprint

Any brand names and product names mentioned in this book are subject to trademark, brand or patent protection and are trademarks or registered trademarks of their respective holders. The use of brand names, product names, common names, trade names, product descriptions etc. even without a particular marking in this work is in no way to be construed to mean that such names may be regarded as unrestricted in respect of trademark and brand protection legislation and could thus be used by anyone.

Cover image: www.ingimage.com

This book is a translation from the original published under ISBN 978-620-6-70755-4.

Publisher:
Sciencia Scripts
is a trademark of
Dodo Books Indian Ocean Ltd. and OmniScriptum S.R.L publishing group

120 High Road, East Finchley, London, N2 9ED, United Kingdom
Str. Armeneasca 28/1, office 1, Chisinau MD-2012, Republic of Moldova, Europe
Printed at: see last page
ISBN: 978-620-7-87897-0

TABLE OF CONTENTS

INTRODUCTION 4

METHODS 6

1.   Type and period of study : 7

2.   Field of study : 7

3.   Study population : 7

   3.1.   Methods : 7
      3.1.1.   Epidemiological data : 7
      3.1.2.   Functional signs : 7
      3.1.3.   Clinical examination data : 7
      3.1.4.   Biological data : 7
      3.1.5.   Imaging data : 7
      3.1.6.   Preoperative section : 8
      3.1.7.   Peroperative section : 8

   3.2.   Judging criteria : 10
      3.2.1.   Occurrence of haemorrhage : 10
      3.2.2.   Other criteria for early surgical morbidity : 11

   3.3.   Statistical analysis : 11

   3.4.   Literature search : 12

RESULTS 13

1.   Descriptive study : 14

   1.1.   Epidemiology : 14
      1.1.1.   Age : 14
      1.1.2.   Gender : 15
      1.1.3.   Background : 15

   1.2.   Diagnostic section : 16
      1.2.1.   Clinical features : 16
      1.2.2.   Biological characteristics : 16
      1.2.3.   Radiological data : 18
      1.2.4.   Therapeutic component : 18
      1.2.5.   Anatomopathological diagnosis : 22
      1.2.6.   Immediate operative follow-up : 22
      1.2.7.   Adjuvant chemotherapy : 27
      1.2.8.   Follow-up : 27

2.   Analytical study: Factors predictive of postoperative hemorrhage : 27

   2.1.   Univariate study : 27
      2.1.1.   Preoperative : 27
      2.1.2.   Intraoperative : 28

2.1.3. Postoperative : 29

2.2. Multivariate study : 30

DISCUSSION...31

1. Results : 32

2. Strengths and weaknesses of the methodology :................................32

3. Postoperative results : 33

3.1. Morbidity :..33

3.1.1. Surgical complications :...34

3.1.2. Medical complications : 44

3.2. Mortality : 44

CONCLUSIONS..47

REFERENCES 53

APPENDICES...62

INTRODUCTION

Cephalic duodeno-pancreatectomy (CPD) is a major operation, but remains the only curative treatment for most tumors of the biliopancreatic crossroads.

In exceptional cases, it is also performed in the event of trauma or chronic pancreatitis.

Improved surgical techniques and postoperative resuscitation have reduced mortality over the past three decades. However, postoperative morbidity remains high, up to 50%. (1)

Among the most frequent complications, hemorrhage following pancreatic fistula represents a particular entity in terms of management and severity.(2). Despite the importance of its impact on morbidity and mortality, few studies have focused specifically on it, particularly in Tunisia.

The main objective of this study was to determine the incidence of post-PCD hemorrhage and to establish its risk factors.

The secondary objectives were to study the characteristics of these haemorrhages, the impact of this complication on 90-day mortality postoperatively and to evaluate the department's practices regarding their management and secondly the overall morbi-mortality of CPB.

METHODS

1. **Type and period of study :**

This is a retrospective, descriptive, monocentric study spanning 13 years, from January 01, 2010 to September 30, 2022, enrolling 32 patients who underwent CPP.

2. **Field of study :**

The study took place in the visceral surgery department of CHU Mongi Slim -la Marsa.

3. **Study population :**

We included in the study all patients who had cephalic duodeno-pancreatectomy regardless of indication, managed at the visceral surgery department of CHU Mongi Slim from January 01, 2010 to September 30, 2022.

We have excluded all unusable and incomplete files.

3.1. Methods :

Data collection was based on hospitalization records, monitoring sheets and anesthesia sheets, all collected on a study sheet (canvas) created for each patient.

This sheet includes :

3.1.1. Epidemiological data :

- Age

- Gender

- Patient's medical and surgical history

3.1.2. Functional signs:

Abdominal pain, Jaundice, Pruritus, Discolored stools, Vomiting, Digestive hemorrhage

3.1.3. Clinical examination data :

General condition, Tenderness to palpation of abdomen, Jaundice, presence of palpable vesicle

3.1.4. Biological data:

Liver workup (look for cytolysis? Cholestasis?) CBC, PT

3.1.5. Image data :

Surgical data :

3.1.6. Preoperative section :

a. Nutritional status:

Assessment of nutritional status prior to CPB is essential to ensure optimal patient management and to prevent postoperative morbidity and mortality.(3)

This assessment was based on weight, height, BMI (Body Mass Index) and measurement of protidemia and albuminemia.(4-6)

b. Preoperative biliary drainage :

Preoperative drainage is designed to combat bile retention, thereby preserving the patient's renal and hepatic function and nutritional status.

Drainage certainly eliminates cholestasis and ensures better patient preparation.

Two types of drainage were used: (7-10).

<u>Endoscopic approach</u>

<u>Percutaneous</u>: Transhepatic under radiological control.

c. Curative antibiotic therapy :

Broad-spectrum antibiotic therapy combining a third-generation cephalosporin + an aminoglycoside + a metronidazole was prescribed in patients with preoperative angiocholitis.

d. Prophylaxis of deep vein thrombosis :

Prevention of deep vein thrombosis after CPD is introduced for all patients as part of the fight against postoperative morbidity and mortality (11-13).

We have used 2 types of deep vein thrombosis prophylaxis:

Mechanical prophylaxis: involving early lifting and mobilization of the patient, as well as the wearing of compression stockings.

Drug prophylaxis: with low-molecular-weight heparin.

This prescription is introduced at least the day before the operation and extended for at least ten days postoperatively.

3.1.7. Peroperative section :

a. Anesthesia and resuscitation : (8,14)

The procedure is performed under general anesthesia, with cardiac and central venous pressure monitoring, and a bladder catheter in place to monitor diuresis.

To prevent the risk of bleeding:

- a reserve of red blood cells and iso-group iso-rhesus PFCs is prepared.

- a central venous catheter is inserted and intraoperative blood loss is quantified using a graduated suction jar.

Antibiotic prophylaxis and administration of sandostatin were systematically used at induction.

b. Surgical technique: (Appendix 1)

Whipple procedure + Child-type assembly : (15-18)

Classically, CPP involves Whipple resection, Child reconstruction and standard lymph node curage.

CPP involves resection of the head of the pancreas, the entire duodenum, the distal part of the stomach and the bile ducts.

The lymph node curage includes resection of the retroportal lamina.

A first approach to the superior mesenteric artery (SMA) is performed for large tumors with doubt about vascular invasion.

The transverse bi-subcostal incision rather than the median approach is generally used.

The first step is exploratory to check that the tumour is respectable.

Investigation and assessment of resectability: (Appendix 1)

The purpose of this time is to assess the possibility of an excision procedure.

We looked for the appearance of the pancreas, the presence of latero-aortic or inter-aotico-caval nodes, the isthmus and body of the gland, and vascular contact with the mesenteric artery and vein, as well as the portal troc.

<u>Exeresis:</u>

Four beats follow one another. The order in which they are performed is not constant.

We begin with cholecystectomy and sectioning of the main bile duct, then the stomach and pancreas, and finish with curage of the retro-portal lamina (Appendix 1).

Restoring pancreatobiliodigestive continuity: Child's approach

This is the most classic technique: the proximal jejunum drains the pancreas, the bile duct and then the stomach:

We start with a pancreatico-digestive anastomosis, in particular the pancreatico-jejunal anastomosis, followed by the terminal hepatico-jejunal anastomosis, 20 to 30 centimetres downstream of the previous one, and finishing with a **gastro-jejunal anastomosis**.

And we end up **draining** it:

Systematic drainage of the peritoneal cavity after CPB is recommended(18) We therefore opted for two Salem catheters or two Redon drains, with or without a corrugated blade, in all patients.

3.2. Judging criteria :

3.2.1. Hemorrhage :

As this is a specific complication, we have included any hemorrhage occurring within 90 days of the operation, whatever its origin (digestive or intraperitoneal), specifying the time and mode of discovery, as well as the chosen therapeutic course.

Bleeding:

A hemorrhage is said to occur **early**: if it occurs within < 24 hours post-operatively.

A hemorrhage is said to be **late** if it occurs > 24 hours postoperatively.

A haemorrhage is said to be **of moderate severity** if :

- blood loss is minimal to moderate, with Hb < 3g/dl.

- Patient's general condition preserved, no treatment required **OR** non-invasive treatment/transfusion of up to three packed red blood cells (RBCs) **OR** endoscopic treatment.

Hemorrhage is said to be **severe** (19) if :

- Massive blood loss and drop in Hb >3g/dl.

- Signs of poor tolerance (hypotension, tachycardia, shock, oliguria)

- Need for transfusion >three RGCs.

- invasive treatment (embolization, interventional angiography, reintervention)

Grade A: Post-CPD hemorrhage is early-onset + inta or extradigestive + moderate in severity.

Grade B: Post-CPD hemorrhage is early-onset + intra- or extradigestive + severe **OR** late-onset + intra- or extradigestive + moderate severity.

Grade C: Post-CPD hemorrhage is late + intra or extradigestive + severe.

3.2.2. Other criteria for early surgical morbidity:

Patients with a complication within 90 days of surgery were included.

Late complications occurring after this period were excluded from this study.

There are two types of early post-operative complications:

a. Specific complications :

Pancreatic fistula: diagnosis is based on amylasemia levels in the drainage fluid (greater than three times normal), as of the third day post-op (20) and persists for three consecutive days.

Biliary fistula: diagnosis based on bile drainage.

Gastric emptying disorder: Essentially gastroparesis, defined by the International Study Group of Pancreatic Surgery (ISGPS) as non-tolerance of solid food from the seventh day onwards, or when the gastric tube is judged to need to be maintained or re-installed after the third day following surgery. (20)

b. Non-specific complications:

Non-specific complications are divided into non-specific *surgical* complications (such as evisceration, wall abscesses, etc.) and *medical* complications (including respiratory infections, urinary tract infections, tare decompensation, etc.).

c. Early operative mortality: defined as death within 90 days of surgery.

3.3. Statistical analysis :

This was a monocentric retrospective study of patients who had undergone cephalic duodeno-pancreatectomy. A pre-established data sheet was used to collect epidemiological, clinical, para-clinical, therapeutic and evolutionary data. Data entry was performed using SPSS 22.0 statistical software.

Qualitative variables were expressed by their frequencies and proportions. Quantitative variables were expressed by their means, standard deviation, confidence interval and relative risk.

Comparisons between two qualitative variables were made using the chi-square test when the conditions for application were met, and the Fisher test in other cases. The comparison between two quantitative variables was ensured by Pearson's and Sperman's correlation tests. The comparison of qualitative variables with quantitative ones was ensured by the parametric Student and ANNOVA tests when normality was assured, and by the non-parametric Wilcoxon and Kruskall Wallis tests in other cases.

A multivariate analysis using logistic regression was performed for variables with a "p" < 0.1 in univariate analysis.

A threshold value for significant quantitative variables was calculated using the ROC curve.

A relationship between variables is considered significant if the correlation coefficient "p" is ≤ 0.05.

3.4. Bibliographic research :

We started by searching for similar theses in the library of the Faculty of Medicine in Tunis.

Literature data were collected by consulting multiple articles on the Internet using the "Pub Med Medline" and "Cochrane Library" websites.

The key words or "Mesh" used were: duodenopancreatectomy, post-CPD hemorrhage, emptying disorder, pancreatic fistula, biliary fistula, early complications, morbi-mortality... and this in two languages, English and French, which finally enabled us to collect the references for this text.

RESULTS

1. Descriptive study :

We collated 32 patients operated on by DPC at the General Surgery Department of Mongi Slim La Marsa Hospital over a 13-year period, from January 01, 2010 to September 30, 2022.

1.1. Epidemiology :

1.1.1. Age :

The average age was 62 years, with extremes of 47 and 75 years, including six patients aged over 70 (2%).

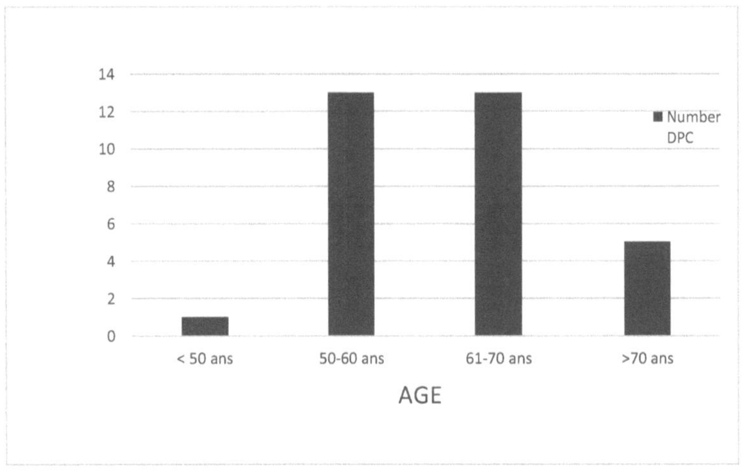

Figure 1 Number of CPDs by age group

1.1.2. Gender :

In our study, 13 men (40%) and 19 women (60%) were involved, giving a sex ratio of 0.68.

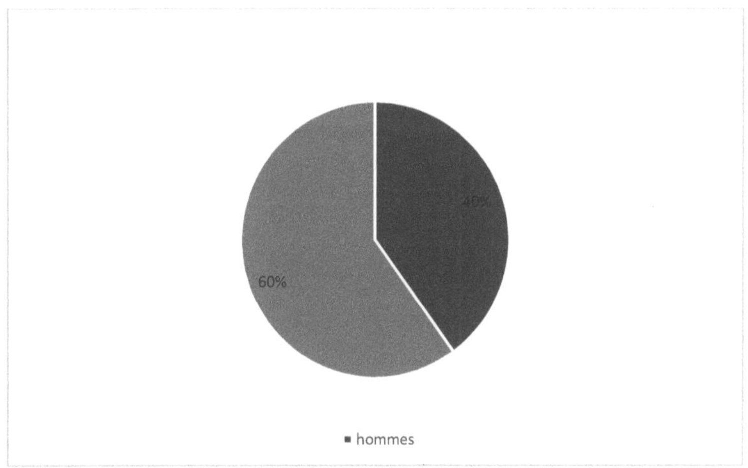

Figure 2 CPD by gender

1.1.3. History:

Eighteen patients (56%) had at least one associated comorbidity.

Nine patients (28%) were hypertensive, thirteen patients (40%) were diabetic and seven patients (21%) were dyslipidemic.

Medical history is detailed in Table 1.

Table I Medical history

Medical history	Number of patients	Frequency
Diabetes	13	41 %
Hypertension	9	28 %
Dyslipidemia	7	22 %
Cardiac pathology	5	16 %
Respiratory pathology	2	6 %
Dysthyroidism	2	6 %

Chronic depression	1	3 %
Anemia	1	3 %

Fifteen patients (46%) had a history of surgery.

Cholecystectomy (25%) and appendectomy (9%) were the most frequent procedures.

Surgical history is detailed in Table 2.

Table II Surgical history

Surgical history	Number of patients	Percentage
Cholecystectomy	8	25%
Appendectomy	3	9 %
Hernia	1	3 %
Hydatid cyst	1	3 %
Hysterectomy+Annexectomy	2	6 %
Uterine fibroma	1	3 %
Total colonoscopy	1	3 %

1.2. Diagnostic section :

1.2.1. Clinical features :

<u>Functional signs :</u>

Abdominal pain was present in 23 patients (71%).

Jaundice was present in 27 patients (84%).

Pruritus was present in 16 patients (50%), with scratching lesions observed in three (13%).

Altered general condition was noted in three patients (9%).

Dark urine was reported in 11 patients (34%).

Discolored stools were reported in 16 patients (50%).

Vomiting was reported in 4 patients (12%).

Digestive haemorrhage of the melena type was observed in two patients (2%).

1.2.2. Biological characteristics :

<u>Liver function tests :</u>

Total bilirubin levels were elevated in 29 patients (96%).

The mean total bilirubin level was 178 µmol/l (14 times normal).

Conjugated bilirubin levels were elevated in 25 patients (78%).

Mean conjugated bilirubin level was 111 µmol/l (11 times normal).

GGT assays were performed in 15 patients, with a mean level of 430IU/l.

(9 times normal).

Transaminases were performed in all our patients.

Cytolysis was noted in 28 patients (88%), with figures ranging from 2 to 11 times normal.

The average TP rate was 88%.

Three patients (9%) had a TP of less than 70%.

<u>Protidemia /Albuminemia :</u>

Protein and albumin levels were measured in only six patients (19%) in our series.

The mean albumin level was 41g/l, with extremes ranging from 30g/l to 84 g/l.

The mean total protein level was 66g/l, with extremes ranging from 53g/l to 76g/L.

<u>Blood count (CBC) :</u>

Mean hemoglobin (Hb) was 11.98 sixteen patients were anemic (50%), with hemoglobin below 12g/dl.

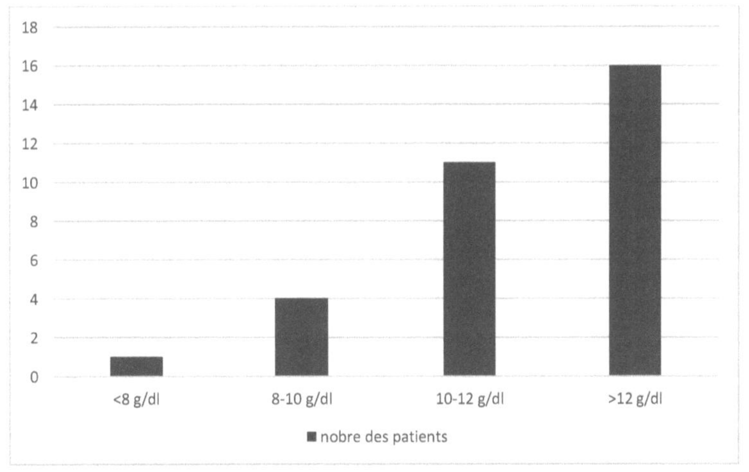

Figure 3 Distribution of patients by hemoglobin level

White blood cell counts averaged around 8225 elements/µl.

Six patients (19%) had hyperleukocytosis.

<u>Renal function :</u>

Creatinemia figures ranged from 21 to 130 µmol/l, with an average of around 62 µmol/l.

Urea values ranged from 2.1 mmol/l to 20 mmol/l, with an average level of 6.3 mmol/l.

Only two patients (6%) developed acute renal failure.

1.2.3. Radiological data :

Abdominal ultrasound and CT scans were performed in all patients.

Biliary dilatation was found in 31 patients (97%).

Dilatation of the Wirsung duct was visualized in 24 patients (77%).

A tumor was visualized on CT in 30 cases (94%), making the preoperative diagnosis.

In 13 cases, the tumor was of the ampulla of Vater (41%), in twelve cases a tumor of the head of the pancreas (37%), including one suspected neuroendocrine tumor, and in five cases a tumor of the lower bile duct (16%).

Four patients (12.5%) presented with angiocholitis (including two patients with tumors of the ampulla of Vater and two patients with tumors of the head of the pancreas).

1.2.4. Therapeutic component :

1.2.4.1. Preoperative management :

a. Medical treatment :

<u>Vitamin k :</u>

Nine patients (28%) had received vitamin K preoperatively.

<u>Antibiotic therapy :</u>

Antibiotic therapy combining a cephalosporin, an aminoglycoside and metronidazole was prescribed in four patients (13%) for acute angiocholitis.

<u>Preoperative transfusion :</u>

Only one patient (3%) received a preoperative transfusion of two packed red blood cells (RBCs).

b. Preoperative biliary drainage :

OFive patients (16%) underwent biliary drainage.

Drainage was performed endoscopically in 4 cases (13%) and percutaneously in a single case (3%).

1.2.4.2. Intraoperative management:

a. Anaesthesia :

All patients underwent general anaesthesia.

b. Antibiotic prophylaxis :

Antibiotic prophylaxis was undertaken in all patients with Augmentin 2g at induction and repeated every four hours if more than four hours.

c. Sandostatin :

Thirteen patients (39%) in our study benefited from intraoperative administration of sandostatin.

d. Surgery :

Approach:

The approach was a bi-subcostal incision in 17 patients (53%) and a midline incision in 14 patients (44%).

Laparoscopic surgery with conversion was chosen in one patient (3%).

Quality of pancreatic parenchyma :

The appearance of the pancreatic parenchyma was described as fibrous in five cases (16%) and soft in a single case (3%).

Wirsung Canal:

The Wirsung duct was dilated (>3 mm) in 23 cases (72%) and thin in seven cases (22%).

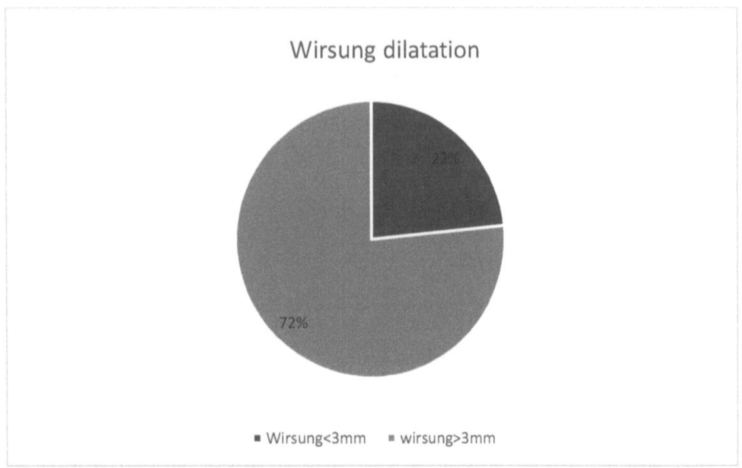

Figure 4 Size of the Wirsung canal

Main bile duct :

The main bile duct was dilated in 30 cases (94%).

Vascular check-up :

Contact with the superior mesenteric vein was noted in three cases (9%) and with the portal vein in three cases (9%).

Gestures :

All patients underwent Whipple CPP with standard lymph node curage. A primary approach to the MSA was performed in only one case. No pyloric PCD was performed.

-Pancreatico-digestive anastomosis:

Pancreatico-digestive anatomy was pancreaticojejunal in all patients.

- Hepaticojejunal anastomosis:

Terminolateral hepaticojejunal anastomosis was performed in all patients.

-Gastrojejunal anastomosis:

Gastrojejunal anastomosis was performed in all patients.

The anastomosis was terminolateral in 30 cases (94%) and laterolateral in two cases (6%).

<u>**Drainage :**</u>

Drainage in contact with the anastomoses was performed in all patients.

Two salem probes combined with a corrugated or Delbet blade were chosen in 11 cases (34%), two salem probes only in 4 cases (13%), and two Redon drains in 8 cases (25%).

<u>**Operating time :**</u>

The average operating time was 362 minutes (6 hours and two minutes), with extremes ranging from 280 minutes (4 hours and 40 minutes) to 520 minutes (8 hours and 40 minutes).

Table III Operating time

	Average	Standard deviation
Operating time	362 MINUTES	82

1.2.4.3. Post-operative management :

The average total hospital stay was 26 days, with extremes ranging from six to 47 days.

Postoperative stay was 13 days, with extremes ranging from four days to 31 days.

Fourteen patients (44%) were hospitalized in the intensive care unit for an average of three days, with extremes ranging from one to eight days.

Table IV Length of hospital stay

	Average	Standard deviation
Total hospital stay	26 days	11.35
Post-operative length of stay	13 days	7.3
Length of stay in intensive care	8 days	2.7

Thromboembolic disease prophylaxis with low-molecular-weight heparin was undertaken for all patients.

A Level 1 analgesic was used in 27 patients (84%) for an average duration of seven days, with extremes ranging from one day to 23 days.

 A Level 2 analgesic was prescribed in 19 patients (59%) for an average of five days, with extremes ranging from one day to 15 days.

Twenty-one patients (66%) were prescribed a Level 3 analgesic for an average of five days, with extremes ranging from one day to 20 days.

Seventeen patients had received sandostatin for an average of nine days, with extremes ranging from three days to 24 days.

1.2.5. Anatomopathological diagnosis :

In 22 cases (69%), the final diagnosis after pathological examination was a malignant lesion, and in only one case (3%) was it chronic pancreatitis.

For the remaining nine cases (28%), the pathology report was not available.

Adenocarcinoma (ADK) was found in 21 patients (66%) and melanoma metastasis was found in only one case (3%).

The location was ampullary in 12 cases (38%), head of pancreas in eight cases (25%) and lower choledochal in 4 cases (13%).

1.2.6. Immediate surgical follow-up:

1.2.6.1. Simple operating sequences :

In our series, thirteen patients (40%) had a simple postoperative course with an average postoperative stay of 13 days.

1.2.6.2. Morbidity :

In our series, nineteen patients suffered postoperative complications, representing an overall morbidity rate of 59%.

Surgical complications accounted for 51% of cases, and medical complications for 7%.

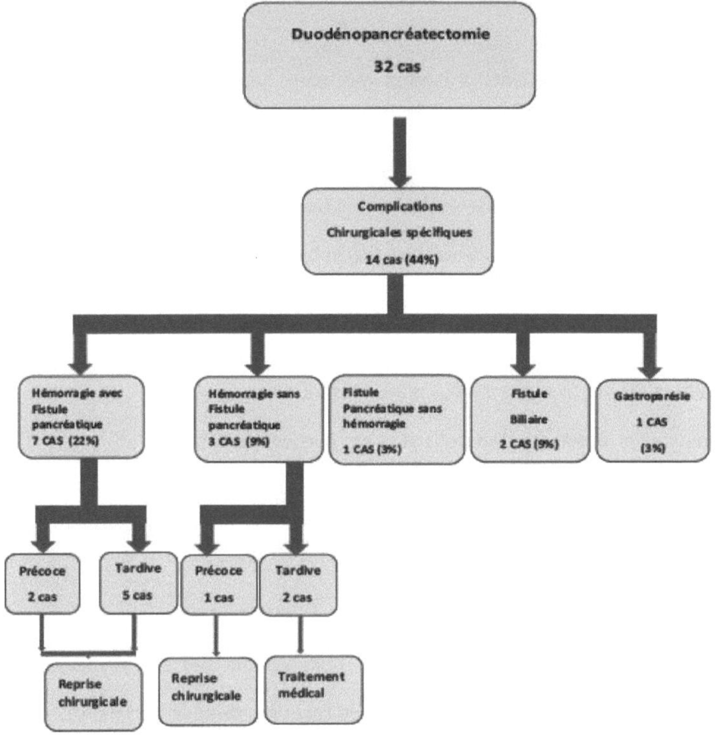

Figure 5 Specific surgical complications

a. Surgical complications :

Sixteen patients (50%) had at least one surgical complication.

a1) Specific surgical complications :

At least one specific surgical complication was noted in 14 patients (44%) in our series.

Hemorrhage:

Ten patients (31%) had experienced postoperative hemorrhage, including seven men and three women.

The average time to onset of hemorrhage was eight days, with extremes ranging from one day to 17 days.

In our series, three patients presented with early hemorrhage and seven with late hemorrhage.

Hemorrhage occurred in four patients with a medical history (mainly diabetics and hypertensives) and in two patients with a surgical history.

Six patients presented with external bleeding in the form of melena.

One patient (3%) had a grade A hemorrhage, two patients (6%) had a grade B hemorrhage and five patients (16%) had a grade C hemorrhage.

The others did not fill in the various grade classifications.

Seven patients developed deglobulization and five went into shock.

Only one patient had an abdominal CT scan, which showed an intra-abdominal effusion.

Six patients were transfused with an average of three packed red blood cells (RBCs), and closely monitored.

Eight patients (25%) underwent reintervention within an average of eight days, with extremes ranging from one day to 13 days. Three patients died after reintervention.

Seven patients were admitted to the intensive care unit, three of whom died.

***Bleeding associated with FP :**

Seven patients had a pancreatic fistula associated with hemorrhage.

Hemorrhage occurred in these patients within an average of four days.

Hemorrhage was early in one patient and late in four.

In all patients, bleeding required reoperation.

***Bleeding without FP:**

Hemorrhage without FP occurred in three patients within an average of seven days.

It was early in one patient and late in two.

Only one patient underwent reoperation.

Table V Intraoperative discovery and procedure during reintervention following haemorrhage

	Number of patients	Gesture
-Release of pancreticjejunal anastomosis + Release of biliodigestive anastomosis -Origin of haemorrhage unidentified	2	Directed fistulization of the biliodigestive anastomosis on kehr drain+suture of the pancreaticojejunal anastomosis.
-Pancreaticojejunal anastomosis release -Origin of haemorrhage unidentified	3	Pancreaticojejunal anastomosis reinforcement + drainage.
Defect at the level of the inferior mesenteric v eine (VMI) + Splenomesara trunk	1	Suture of venous defect + reconfection of pancreaticojejunal anastomosis.
Abdominal wall hematoma	1	Surgical hemostasis.
Digestive bleeding from the hepatic artery	1	Elective hemostasis of the hepatic artery and totalization of the pancreatectomy.

<u>Pancreatic fistula:</u>

A pancreatic fistula was discovered in eight patients (25%) with a mean postoperative delay of six days, ranging from one day to 12 days.

A pancreatic fistula without bleeding was diagnosed in just one patient.

The diagnosis of pancreatic fistula was retained after amylase determination of the drained fluid in six patients.

Abdominal CT scans were performed on all patients.

Seven of the pancreatic fistulas were graded Grade B and only one was graded Grade C.

All patients received medical treatment.

Antibiotic therapy was initiated in seven cases for an average duration of ten days (with a minimum of two days and a maximum of 16 days).

Sandostatin was administered to six patients.

Three fistulas were misdirected, one of which was complicated by generalized peritonitis.

Six patients underwent reoperation within an average of eight days postoperatively , with extremes ranging from four days to 16 days.

We opted for reconfection or reinforcement of the pancreaticojejunal anastomosis and cleansing with drainage in five cases, and totalization of the pancreatectomy in a single case.

Four cases had a good outcome, and two were fatal.

Biliary fistula :

A biliary fistula was discovered in three patients (9%) with an average postoperative delay of four days, with extremes ranging from one day to eight days .

The fistula was well directed in all three cases.

An abdominal CT scan was performed in only one case.

In two cases, the patient was placed under close surveillance and given antibiotics for an average of eight days.

In no case did we have to resort to a reoperation.

Gastroparesis:

Only one patient (3%) presented with an emptying disorder revealed by vomiting.

The patient was put on Primperan and a nasogastric tube with good progression.

a2) Other specific surgical complications :

Only one patient presented with acute pancreatitis complicated by pancreatic abscess.

a 3) Non-specific surgical complications :

In our series, five patients (16%) suffered from non-specific surgical complications, including two cases of evisceration (6%) and two cases of liver abscesses (6%).

b. Medical complications :

Eight patients (25%) had one or more non-specific medical complications:

Four patients (12%) had a urinary tract infection, three patients (9%) had a respiratory infection, three patients (9%) had decompensated heart disease, and one patient (3%) had acute renal failure.

1.2.6.3. Mortality :

The early post-operative mortality rate (i.e. within 90 days of surgery) was 34% (11 patients).

The patients who died were five men (16%) and six women (19%).

The average age of the deceased patients was 67, with extremes ranging from 52 to 75 years.

Ten patients (31%) died as a result of postoperative complications.

Seven patients (22%) died as a result of a specific surgical complication:

Three patients (9%) died from postoperative haemorrhage.

 Two patients (6%) died following pancreatic fistula without associated hemorrhage.

Two patients (6%) died from biliary fistula.

Only one patient (3%) died as a result of a medical complication: decompensation of ischemic heart disease.

1.2.7. Adjuvant chemotherapy :

Five patients received adjuvant chemotherapy for pancreatic head ADK.

1.2.8. Follow-up:

Twenty-one patients (66%) attended the Mongi Slim outpatient surgery clinic for postoperative follow-up.

The average total number of consultations was eight, with extremes ranging from a single consultation to 20 consultations.

Five patients (16%) continued their post-chemotherapy follow-up at the oncology outpatient clinic (Salah Azaiz and Ariana), with an average of five consultations.

2. Analytical study: Predictive factors of postoperative hemorrhage :

2.1. Uni-varied study:

In order to determine the predictive factors for the occurrence of postoperative hemorrhage, we carried out a univariate study of all pre-, intra- and postoperative data:

2.1.1. Preoperative:

With regard to epidemiological factors, male gender was significantly more frequent in the group in which a hemorrhagic complication occurred (p=0.045). On the other hand, age, patient medical and surgical history, vitamin K administration and biliary drainage were not significantly associated with post-CPD hemorrhage.

The various parameters are summarized in Table 5.

Table VI Preoperative predictive factors for post-CPD hemorrhage

Preoperative data	No bleeding %	Hemorrhage %	P
Male gender	6 (18%)	7 (21%)	**0.045**
Age			0.58
Medical history	13 (40%)	4 (13%)	0.18
Surgical history	11 (34%)	2 (6%)	0.74
Vitamin K	6 (18%)	3 (9%)	0.42
Biliary drainage	3 (9%)	0	0.43

2.1.2. Intraoperative:

Operative time was significantly associated with post-CPD hemorrhage (p=0.017).

Wirsung diameter, bile duct dilatation and parenchymal quality, on the other hand, did not appear to significantly influence the occurrence of this complication.

Construction of the ROC curve for operating time showed a threshold of 395 minutes.

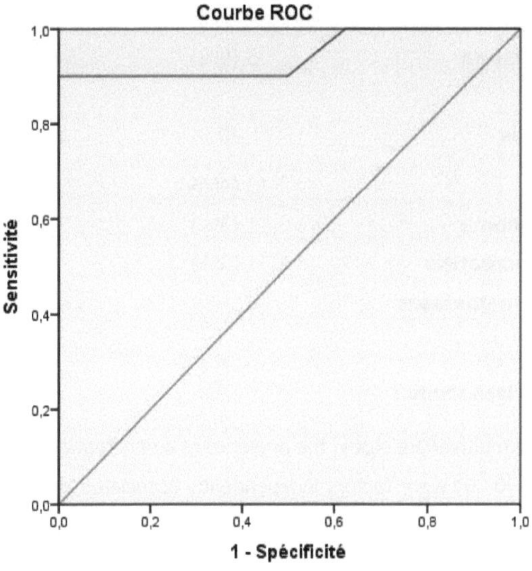

Figure 6 ROC curve representing the best predictive threshold for the occurrence of postoperative bleeding .

Table VII Intraoperative predictors of post-PCD hemorrhage

Intraoperative data	No bleeding %	Hemorrhage %	P
Operating time	16 (50%)	10 (31%)	**0.017**
Wirsung fine diameter	5 (16%)	2 (6%)	0.54
Friable pancreatic parenchyma	1 (3%)	0	0.31

2.1.3. Post-operative:

Postoperatively, the presence of a pancreatic fistula has been validated as a predisposing factor for the occurrence of post-PCD hemorrhage .

Table VIII Postoperative predictive factors for post-PCD hemorrhage

Postoperative data	No bleeding %	Hemorrhage e	P

		%	
Pancreatic fistula	3 (9%)	5 (15%)	**0.037**
Gastroparesis	0	1 (3%)	0.33
Histology:	13 (40%)	7 (22%)	0.59
-Adenocarcinoma	1 (3%)	0	
-chronic pancreatitis	1 (3%)	0	
-melanoma metastases			

2.2. Multivariate study :

After performing a multivariate study, the presence of a pancreatic fistula (p=0.021) and operative time (p=0.00) were factors independently associated with the occurrence of early or late post-CPD hemorrhage.

Table IX Predictive factors for post-CPD hemorrhage in multivariate analysis

Data	**No bleeding** %	**Hemorrhage** %	**P**
Pancreatic fistula	3 (9%)	5 (15%)	0.021
Operating time	16 (50%)	10 (31%)	0.000
Male gender	6 (18%)	7 (21%)	0.087

DISCUSSION

1. Reminder of results:

Our study included 32 patients who underwent CPP.

The mean age of these patients was 62 years, with extremes ranging from

 47 to 75 years of age. The majority were women, with a sex ratio of 0.68.

The final diagnosis after pathological examination was malignant in 22 patients (69%), and chronic pancreatitis in just one (3%).

Malignant lesions include adenocarcinoma in 66% of cases and pancreatic metastases in 3%.

The location was ampullary in 34% of cases, the head of the pancreas in 22% and the lower bile duct in 9%.

Whipple CPP with standard lymph node curage was performed in all cases. A primary approach to the MSA was performed in only one case.

Mean operating time was 362 minutes (6 hours), with extremes ranging from 280 minutes (4 hours 40 minutes) to 520 minutes (8 hours 40 minutes).

The morbidity rate was of 54 %.

Forty-three percent of our series developed at least one specific surgical complication distributed as follows:

postoperative hemorrhage in 31% of cases, hemorrhage associated with pancreatic fistula in 22% of cases, not associated with pancreatic fistula in 9% of cases

 Isolated pancreatic fistula occurred in 25% of cases, biliary fistula in 9%, gastroparesis in 3% and pancreatic abscess in 3%.

In our series, the mortality rate operated early was 34%. Sixteen percent were men and 19% were women. The patients who died had an average age of 67, with extremes ranging from 52 to 75 years.

For postoperative hemorrhage, three factors were significantly associated with the occurrence of this complication: male gender, presence of a pancreatic fistula and operative time > 395 minutes (6h35 min).

In a multivariate study, the presence of a pancreatic fistula and an operating time > 395 minutes (6h35 min) were selected as independent predisposing factors to hemorrhage.

2. Strengths and weaknesses of the methodology :

All our patients were operated on using the same surgical technique, i.e. Whipple CPP with standard lymph node curage, thus reducing selection and performance bias.

Monocentricity was one of the main limitations of our study, as it represented a selection bias.

We tried to analyze most of the factors predictive of the occurrence of postoperative hemorrhage reported in the literature, but the retrospective nature of the study and the absence of optimal control of the data collected also represented an obstacle to the smooth running of our study, given that some files lacked precision or certain essential data.

Finally, the small sample size made it impossible to carry out

Analytical study impossible for some factors.

3. Postoperative results:

3.1. Morbidity :

Despite improvements in surgical techniques over the past thirty years, morbidity associated with CPP remains high, as confirmed by our study.

Indeed, depending on the series, it varies between 50% and 55% in the Tunisian series (23-25).

Table X Postoperative morbidity in Tunisian series

series	Year	Workforce	Morbidity rate
Makni(23)	2005	60	52%
Baccar(24)	2014	69	54%
ATC monograph (25)	2016	448	53%
Hamdi Kbir(25)	2018	44	50%
Our series	2022	32	59%

It is lower in international series, ranging from 25% to 45% (26-29).

Table XI Postoperative morbidity in international series

series	Year	Workforce	Morbidity rate
Yang(26)	2005	62	44%

MORIN(27)	2006	79	45%
D.Y Greenblatt et al(28)	2011	4945	27%
J.L Cameron(29)	2014	2000	45%
Our series	2022	32	59%

In our series, the overall morbidity rate was around 59%, which is comparable to Tunisian series and higher than in international series.

Medical complications accounted for 7% and surgical complications for 51%.

Non-specific surgical complications were found in 15% of patients, and at least one specific surgical complication in 43%.

3.1.1. Surgical complications :

3.1.1.1. Postoperative hemorrhage:

Hemorrhage post CPP occurs in 2% to 16% of cases.(30) (31) and is responsible for 11% to 38% of the mortality rate. It is considered an independent factor in mortality (19).

In our series, ten patients (31%) had experienced post-CPD hemorrhage, including seven men and three women.

Seven patients were admitted to the intensive care unit, three of whom died.

The average time to onset of hemorrhage was eight days, with extremes ranging from one day to 17 days.

In our series, two patients presented with early hemorrhage (<24 hours) and six with late hemorrhage (>24 hours).

The International Study Group of Pancreatic Surgery (ISGPS) has defined three grades of severity: A, B and C, based on the time to onset of bleeding, its location and severity (19).

In our series, one patient presented with grade A hemorrhage, two patients presented with grade B hemorrhage and five patients presented with grade C hemorrhage.

We must therefore be vigilant in the face of this type of complication, and envisage rigorous monitoring in the surgical care unit, based on the identification of factors predictive of its occurrence.

a. Predisposing factors :

Several factors are incriminated in the occurrence of postoperative hemorrhage:

*Preoperative factors

Several studies have shown that males are more exposed to the risk of bleeding (32,33).

This is consistent with our series. Indeed, of the ten patients with post-CPD hemorrhage, seven were male.

Advanced age(32) and the patient's condition, particularly if hypertensive (34)malnourished, obese (35) or with a history of digestive surgery(36) were also identified as risk factors for post-CPD hemorrhage.

Smoking appears to be a protective factor in some series. Two hypotheses have been put forward in this respect: the vasoconstrictive effect of nicotine on the vessels, and the fibrosing action of tobacco on the pancreatic parenchyma, thus reducing the risk of FPs known for their erosive potential.(34).

In our study, age and the patient's medical and surgical history were not significantly associated with hemorrhage.

Data on the patient's nutritional status, BMI and smoking habits are not available.

These data should be sought out and recorded in the patient's file, so that the benefit/risk ratio of CPD can be assessed according to the patient's profile, and so that candidates for CPD can be better prepared.

*Intraoperative factors:

Surgical expertise is a determining factor in the occurrence of post-CPD hemorrhage. Careful vascular suturing and anastomosis is the only way to reduce the risk of bleeding.

For intraoperative findings, a thin diameter of the Wirsung appears to be a risk factor for the occurrence of hemorrhage in the literature (37).

Soft pancreatic tissue and significant intraoperative blood loss are known risk factors for the occurrence of pancreatic fistula, and may therefore indirectly lead to hemorrhage, but these factors have not been validated as independent risk factors.(35).

In our series, a fine Wirsung diameter was not associated with a high risk of haemorrhage.

Our study lacks data on pancreatic tissue quality and quantification of intraoperative blood loss.

Several studies have established a causal link between long operative time and the occurrence of post-CPD complications in general(38). However, the relationship between operative time and the occurrence of post-CPD hemorrhage, in particular, remains poorly studied in the literature.

In our study, an operating time > 395 minutes (6h35 min) was selected as a predictive factor for the occurrence of hemorrhage.

This can be explained by the fact that a long operative time is generally synonymous with operative difficulty due to vascular relationships. Long operative time is also usually associated with an increased risk of infection, which in itself represents a risk factor for the occurrence of post-CPD hemorrhage.

*Postoperative factors:

Several studies have shown that the occurrence of infection, intra-abdominal abscess (especially if misdirected) or pancreatic fistula(35,36) is a risk factor for post-CPD hemorrhage.

Our study corroborates the findings of the literature regarding the increased risk and severity of bleeding in the presence of pancreatic fistula.

The pathophysiological explanation is uncertain: erosion of vessel walls by pancreatic fluid is the most commonly described.

b. Origin of hemorrhage :

Post-CPD hemorrhage may initially reveal itself as "sentinel bleeding"(39,40)This consists of moderate bleeding diagnosed clinically (externalized bleeding) or biologically (loss of one hemoglobin point between D1 and D3), preceding a major hemorrhagic event or even a state of shock, hence the importance of close monitoring to detect it at an early stage.

Hemorrhage can be either intraperitoneal or digestive in origin.

Bleeding may follow loosening of the gastro-jejunal or pancreatic-gastric anastomosis(41) ,an ulcer or pseudoaneurysm(42).

Hemorrhage may also be secondary to excision of the gastroduodenal artery(43)celiac trunk, superior mesenteric artery, hepatic artery or splenic artery.(39,41)

In our series, hemorrhage was secondary to loosening of the pancreatico-jejunal anastomosis in seven cases, injury to the inferior mesenteric vein in a single case, and injury to the hepatic artery in a single case.

In two cases, the origin of the bleeding was not identified.

c. Management of post-CPD hemorrhage:

<u>Endoscopic treatment :</u>

Digestive origin is suspected if the patient presents melena or hematemesis.

If digestive hemorrhage (early or late) is suspected, endoscopy is performed for both diagnostic and therapeutic purposes(44).

Once the patient has been hemodynamically stabilized, endoscopy is used to localize the bleeding and perform a hemostasis procedure.

The disadvantage of this method is that it lacks sensitivity. Indeed, the literature reports that it may present false positives, and that the real origin of the bleeding may not be detected, resulting in diagnostic and therapeutic delay.(45)

If the bleeding is localized and the hemostasis procedure was successful, an endoscopic check-up should be scheduled; if this is unsuccessful, laparotomy is performed.

In our series, no patient received endoscopic treatment.

In fact, the therapeutic contribution of endoscopy is mainly in cases of pancreatico-gastric anastomosis, whereas in our study all patients had a pancreatico-jejunal anastomosis.

<u>Radiological treatment :</u>

 After stabilization of the patient, an injected angioscan must precede any therapeutic decision, as it allows us to localize the hemorrhage (44,46).

Conservative treatment should be preferred wherever possible.

Interventional radiology is most often indicated for late hemorrhage in hemodynamically stable patients.

This treatment consists of arterial embolization, combined, of course, with resuscitation measures. (47).

This proven technique is appreciated for its minimally invasive nature, rapidity, low morbidity and hospital stay, and a success rate of between 72% and 100%. (48).

However, it does have its limitations: it is possible to miss the origin of the bleed if it is venous, diffuse or intermittent; as well as technical difficulty, especially if bleeding occurs from the stump of the gastroduodenal artery, hence the advantage of leaving a long stump intraoperatively. (45)

In our series, no patient underwent radiological treatment.

<u>Surgical treatment :</u>

There are a number of causes for post-CPD reintervention. Haemorrhage is the leading cause of post-CPD reintervention, accounting for 68% of cases. (30,45)

Despite advances in non-invasive techniques, revision is often unavoidable when bleeding is associated with septic complications, the patient is hemodynamically unstable, and conservative treatment has failed or is unavailable.

Due to the unavailability of non-invasive means , reintervention was performed in seven of our patients (with an average delay of 8 days), which may partly explain the high mortality rate associated with post-CPD hemorrhage in our series.

Nevertheless, an angioscanner is recommended to identify the origin of the hemorrhage and to determine the indication for laparotomy(46).

During revision, the procedure performed depends on the origin of the bleeding, hence the need for rigorous inspection of the celiac trunk, gastroduodenal artery, superior mesenteric artery, portal tract, portal vein and its branches, and pancreticojejunal, hepatojejunal and gastrojejunal anastomoses.(37).

Hemostasis should be performed if the source of bleeding is identified, and the drainage repositioned.

Among the principal procedures performed during laparotomy reported in the literature (37,49) include :

-Suturing a pancreatic parenchymal lesion

-Suture of hemorrhagic sites in pancreaticojejunal, hepatojejunal or gastrojejunal anastomoses.

-Suture of the injured artery (gastroduodenal, mesocolic, hepatic, splenic, etc.)

-Suture of injured vein (portal vein, branches of superior mesenteric vein, etc.)

-Suturing a wall wound

-Abdominal packing: is a temporary measure when bleeding cannot be stopped, pending stabilization of the patient and correction of coagulation disorders, before proceeding with a second laparotomy. (49).

In our series :

-Three patients presented with loosening of the pancreaticojejunal anastomosis requiring reinforcement of the pancreaticojejunal anstomosis with drainage.

-Two patients presented with both a loose pancreaticojejunal anastomosis and a loose biliodigestive anastomosis requiring directed fistulization of the biliodigestive anastomosis with suturing of the pancreaticojejunal anastomosis.

-Only one patient had a venous defect in the inferior mesenteric vein and splenomesenteric trunk requiring suturing.

-Only one patient presented with a wall hematoma requiring surgical hemostasis.

Totalization of the pancreatectomy may be necessary in certain cases, but is associated with a high mortality rate ranging from 24% to 80%, as well as significant morbidity, notably diabetes that is difficult to control and impairs the patient's quality of life.(46).

In our series, a patient presented with severe hemorrhage originating from the hepatic artery, the course of action was to perform hepatic artery hemostasis with totalization of the pancreatectomy.

In 10% of cases, the origin of the haemorrhage cannot be identified during laparotomy, resulting in massive blood loss and multivisceral failure followed by death (37,49).

3.1.1.2. Pancreatic fistula (PF):

This is the most serious complication of CPP.

The incidence of pancreatic fistula varies between 1% and 36%. (50). Pancreatic fistula is responsible for 70% of mortality rates, due to the septic and hemorrhagic complications associated with it(51).

It is due to disunion of the pancreatico-digestive anastomosis.

In our series, PF was discovered in eight patients (25%), two of whom died. FP was discovered with an average post-PCD delay of six days.

The 'ISGPF (International Study Group of Pancreatic Fistula) defined pancreatic fistula in 2005 as the existence of fluid leakage from a drain (placed intraoperatively or postoperatively) from the third day post-op, associated with an amylase level greater than three times the normal serum level (20,52).

Three grades have been defined:

Grade A: Asymptomatic, requiring no specific therapeutic action.

Grade B: General condition preserved, no signs of severe sepsis or major bleeding, medical treatment recommended.

Grade C: life-threatening, requiring resuscitative measures and additional surgical drainage procedures.

a. FP processing:

Once the diagnosis of FP has been confirmed, treatment appropriate to the grade should be started as soon as possible.

Grade A: good clinical tolerance, spontaneous dry-off possible, so conservative treatment and per os feeding are recommended. Some studies have demonstrated the value of sondostatins in reducing the duration of evolution of these PF (53,54).

Grade B: Conservative treatment is also recommended for this type of fistula:

-Nasogastric tube / total parenteral nutrition.

-Appropriate antibiotic therapy for drainage samples is recommended.

Endoscopic or ultrasound-guided drainage, if unsuccessful, proceed to surgery (55).

Grade C: One reintervention (54,56) is the rule in the following situations:

- a hemorrhage that cannot be treated by radioguided embolization

-peritonitis

-an abscess inaccessible to percutaneous drainage.

The rate of reintervention following pancreatic fistula varies between 5% and 39% depending on the study, with a mortality rate of around 39%. (57).

The details are controversial.

Some teams prefer to preserve the pancreas, opting for anastomosis with drainage or fistulization.

However, this attitude exposes us to a significant hemorrhagic and septic risk, which could force us to re-intervene.

Other teams recommend immediate totalization of the pancreatectomy, at the risk of permanent diabetes that is difficult to control(58).

In our series, out of a total of eight patients with VT, seven were graded Grade B and only one was graded Grade C.

The absence of Grade A in our series may be explained, in part, by the fact that amylase assay of drained fluid is not routinely performed.

All patients received medical treatment.

Antibiotic therapy was initiated in seven cases for an average duration of ten days.

Three fistulas were misdirected, one of which was complicated by generalized peritonitis.

Seven patients underwent reoperation within an average of eight days.

We opted for reconfection or reinforcement of the anastomosis combined with flushing and drainage in six cases, and totalization of the pancreatectomy in just one case.

b. FP risk factors :

<u>Patient-related factors</u> : (59,60)

-The masculine gender

-BMI >25

-Weight loss > 3kg in the six months prior to surgery.

However, diabetes appears to be a protective factor against PF.

<u>Pathology-related risk factors :</u>

Cancer of the duodenum, choledochus, ampulloma and tumors of the

endocrine diseases are more likely to cause FP than adenocarcinoma or chronic or obstructive pancreatitis. (61).

<u>Intraoperative risk factors :</u>

-The soft consistency of pancreatic parenchyma is a predisposing factor for PF, which explains the low rate of PF if there is a history of chronic or obstructive pancreatitis; a fatty pancreas, as opposed to a fibrous one, is more prone to PF (62).

 - Wirsung duct diameter < 3 mm (63).

-Type of anastomosis: Pancreaticojejunal anastomosis appears to be more conducive to PF than pancreaticogastric anastomosis (64).

This may be explained by the fact that the activity of pancreatic enzymes is partially inhibited by gastric acidity, which makes secretion

less deleterious for the anastomosis.

In addition, the richly vascularized gastric wall provides excellent vascularization for the anastomosis.

In our series, six patients presented with a dilated Wirsung duct out of eight patients with VT.

3.1.1.3. Biliary fistula :

The incidence of post-CPD biliary fistula varies between 3% and 8%.

It is caused by disruption of the hepaticojejunal anastomosis, and its diagnosis is based on the presence of a bilirubin level at least three times that of normal bilirubinemia in the abdominal drainage fluid, from the third postoperative day onwards (65).

In the majority of cases, this is a well-tolerated complication, which is drained by the drainage left at the end of the operation, with good progress.

However, it can also lead to biliary collection or peritonitis, requiring radiological or surgical drainage.

Reoperation to repair or intubate the anastomosis with a Kehr drain may therefore be necessary. (65)

Intubation via a percutaneous trans-hepatic approach may also be considered.

In our series, a biliary fistula was found in only three patients (9%). It was well directed in all three cases.

In two cases, the patient was placed under close surveillance and given antibiotics for an average of eight days.

In no case did we have to resort to a reoperation.

Two patients died.

Several studies have reported that advanced age, obesity, hypoalbuminemia and association with other post-CPD complications (hemorrhage and pancreatic fistula) are the main risk factors for the occurrence of biliary fistula (65).

3.1.1.4. Gastroparesis:

It was defined by the International Study Group of Pancreatic Surgery (ISGPS) in 2007 as non-tolerance of solid food from the seventh day onwards, or when it is deemed that the gastric tube must be maintained or rested after the third day following surgery (66)

It is the most frequent complication after CPP, occurring in 40 to 57% of patients operated on (67,68). It corresponds to a delay in gastric emptying without any detectable organic mechanical obstacle, resulting in a delay in the resumption of oral feeding.

Gastroparesis is rarely life-threatening, but it is responsible for impairment of the patient's quality of life and a high readmission rate(69).

It significantly increases the cost and duration of hospitalization by 50%.

In our series, only one patient presented with gastroparesis, which progressed well under medical treatment.

a. Predictive factors for gastroparesis :

Preparatory course :

-Age >75 (70)

-Diabetes (71)

- overweight (BMI>25 kg/m2)(72)

Intraoperative:

Several studies have shown that **pylorus-sparing CPP** is more likely to cause gastroparesis than Whipple CPP.

Several authors support the hypothesis that pylorospasm is responsible for the onset of gastroparesis, and therefore opt for the Whipple technique to prevent this complication, as it associates antrectomy.(73)

With regard to the modalities of surgical reconstruction, several trials and meta-analyses have suggested that there is no significant difference between pancreaticogastric and pancreaticojejunal anastomosis (74,75).

<u>Postoperative:</u>

The coexistence of other complications, notably **pancreatic fistulas** and **intra-abdominal abscesses,** increases the incidence of gastroparesis (76).

b. Processing :

Treatment of gastroparesis includes dietary measures and the administration of standard prokinetics such as metoclopramide or domperidone.

As a second-line treatment, intravenous erythromycin may be considered (77).

In our study, only one patient presented with gastroparesis revealed by vomiting.

He was put on metoclopramide and a nasogastric tube with good progression.

3.1.2. Medical complications :

The rate of medical complications varies from series to series, and can reach 8%. (78).

In the series by Han et al(79) medical complications were dominated by respiratory infections (4%) and the onset of diabetes mellitus (2%).

In the Schmidt series(78)series, cardiorespiratory complications were around 15% and surgical site infections around 5%.

In our series, the rate of medical complications was higher than in international series, reaching 25%.

These complications were essentially infectious (12% urinary tract infections and 9% respiratory infections) or the decompensation of a defect (9%).

3.2. Mortality:

When duodeno-pancreatectomy was first described in the 60s and 70s, it was associated with a very high mortality rate of up to 25%. (80).

Mortality has fallen considerably in recent years, and currently stands at 5% to 8%. (81).

There is an indisputable relationship between the team's experience in pancreatic surgery and the quality of the post-operative follow-up, and it follows that in centers with a high volume of operations, the mortality rate is even lower, at around 1.5%. (29,80).

In Tunisian series, post-CPD mortality remains high:

18% in the series by Hamdi Kbir et al, 17% in the series by Baccar et al, 8% in the series by Makni et al and finally 16% in the Tunisian series by L'association tunisienne de chirurgie (ATC) in 2016.

In our series, the mortality rate was even higher, at 34%.

This can be explained by the comoribidities presented by the patients and the advanced nature of the tumors operated on in our department.

In fact, the causes of death are multiple and interlinked.

 Of course, post-operative surgical complications remain the most common cause, but the terrain and the balance of morbidities must not be overlooked.

An advanced age in excess of 75 years is a risk factor for mortality, according to several studies (85,86).

In our series, the patients who died had an average age of 67, with extremes ranging from 52 to 75 years.

The presence of comorbidities, mainly cardiorespiratory (hypertension, obstructive lung disease), renal insufficiency, dementia, undernutrition and hypoalbuminemia, as well as neoadjuvant treatment, are factors with a poor prognosis (28,85).

In our series, 56% had at least one associated comorbidity.

(Of which 28% were hypertensive and 40% diabetic)

Finally, the surgeon's experience (79) and the selection criteria for patients undergoing CPD also remain determining factors in postoperative morbidity and mortality (58).

Indeed, specialization in pancreatic surgery can lead to improved results.

Specific complications, in particular postoperative hemorrhage and fistulas, are predictive of mortality, especially if they involve reoperation (which is in itself a risk factor). (84, 87,88).

Reintervention is associated with a mortality rate ranging from 23 to 67%. (89).

In our series, only one patient died as a result of a medical complication: tare decompensation.

Thirty-one percent of patients died as a result of a specific surgical complication: 9% as a result of postoperative haemorrhage and 13% as a result of pancreatic or biliary fistula.

Table XII Postoperative mortality in Tunisian series

series	Year	Workforce	Mortality rate
Makni (23)	2005	60	8
Baccar (24)	2014	79	17
ATC Monograph(82)	2016	448	16
Hamdi Kbir(25)	2018	44	18
Our series	2022	32	34

Table XIII Postoperative mortality in international series

series	Year	Workforce	Mortality rate
J.S. Hill et al.(83)	2010	5715	6%
D.Y Greenblatt et a(28)	2011	4945	3%
J.L Cameron(29)	2014	2000	1%
Narayanan et al(84)	2016	551	4%
Our series	2022	32	34%

CONCLUSIONS

Cephalic duodeno-pancreatectomy (CPD) is a high-risk surgery, but remains the only curative treatment for certain tumors of the bilio-pancreatic junction.

It may also be indicated in rare cases of chronic pancreatitis or in the context of trauma.

Improved surgical techniques and resuscitation have reduced mortality rates over the years, but the postoperative morbidity rate remains high, at around 50%.

The most frequent postoperative complications include hemorrhage associated with biliary fistulas, isolated hemorrhage, biliary and pancreatic fistulas, and gastroparesis.

Post-CPD hemorrhage is poorly studied in the literature, despite the fact that it is most often fatal.

The main objective of this study was to determine the rate of immediate morbidity and mortality associated with this procedure in general, and postoperative hemorrhage in particular, as well as to identify the risk factors for its occurrence.

We therefore conducted a retrospective study including all patients who had undergone CPD at the Visceral Surgery Department of CHU Mongi Slim over a 12-year period, from January 01, 2010 to September 30, 2022.

Data relating to the immediate postoperative period were collected on a data collection form and then statistically analyzed.

Our series included 32 patients, divided into 13 men (41%) and 19 women (60%), giving a sex ratio of 0.68.

The average age was 62, with extremes of 47 and 75.

In terms of clinical data, abdominal pain was present in 23 patients, jaundice in 27 and pruritus in 16.

Altered general condition was noted in three patients.

With regard to biological data, bilirubin levels were elevated in 29 patients (mean 178 µmol/l). Sixteen patients were anemic (50%), with hemoglobin below 12g/dl. The mean albumin level was 41g/l.

All patients underwent preoperative abdominal ultrasound and CT scans. A tumor was visualized by CT in 30 cases (94%), making the preoperative diagnosis.

The final diagnosis after anatomical-pathological examination was adenocarcinoma (ADK) in 21 cases (66%), metastasis of melanoma in one case (3%) and chronic pancreatitis in one case (3%).

All patients underwent Whipple CPP with standard lymph node dissection, and only one underwent primary approach to the MSA. No pyloric PCD was performed.

The approach was a bicostal incision in 17 cases (53%) and a midline incision in 14 cases (44%).

Laparoscopic surgery with conversion was chosen in only one case (3%).

The Wirsung duct was dilated (>3 mm) in 23 cases (72%).

Pancreatico-digestive anatomy was pancreaticojejunal in 30 cases (94%).

The average operating time was 362 minutes (6 hours and two minutes), with extremes ranging from 280 minutes (4 hours and 40 minutes) to 520 minutes (8 hours and 40 minutes).

The postoperative mortality rate was 34%.

Ten patients (31%) died as a result of postoperative complications.

Seven patients (22%) died as a result of a specific surgical complication:

Three patients (9%) died from postoperative haemorrhage.

 Two patients (6%) died following pancreatic fistula.

Two patients (6%) died from biliary fistula.

Only one patient (3%) died as a result of a medical complication: tare decompensation.

In our study, 19 patients suffered postoperative complications, representing an overall morbidity rate of 59%.

Medical complications occurred in 7% of cases, and surgical complications in 51%.

In our series, five patients (16%) had non-specific surgical complications and 14 patients (44%) had at least one specific surgical complication.

Ten patients (32%) had experienced postoperative hemorrhage, including seven men and three women.

The average time to onset of bleeding was eight days (with extremes ranging from one day to 17 days).

Five patients had a pancreatic fistula associated with hemorrhage.

One patient had a grade A hemorrhage, two patients had a grade B hemorrhage and five patients had a grade C hemorrhage.

Hemorrhage was due to loosening of the pancreatic-gastric anastomosis in seven cases, injury to the inferior mesenteric vein in one case and injury to the hepatic artery in one case.

Six patients were transfused with an average of three packed red blood cells, and closely monitored.

Eight patients underwent reintervention within an average of eight days (with extremes ranging from one day to 13 days). Three patients died after reintervention.

The univariate study showed that male gender(p=0.045), operative time(p=0.017) and the presence of a pancreatic fistula(p=0.037) were predisposing factors for the occurrence of post-PCD hemorrhage.

The construction of the ROC curve found a threshold of 395 minutes.

In a multivariate study, the presence of a pancreatic fistula and the duration of the operation were independently associated with the occurrence of hemorrhage.

A pancreatic fistula was discovered in eight patients (25%) with a mean postoperative delay of six days.

Seven of the FPs were classified as Grade B and only one as Grade C.

All patients received medical treatment.

Antibiotic therapy was initiated in seven cases for an average duration of ten days.

Three fistulas were misdirected, one of which was complicated by generalized peritonitis.

Seven patients underwent reoperation within an average of eight days postoperatively.

We opted for reconfection or reinforcement of the pancreaticojejunal anastomosis and cleansing with drainage in five cases, and totalization of the pancreatectomy in a single case.

Four cases had a good outcome, and two were fatal.

Biliary fistulas were discovered in three patients (9%) with a mean postoperative delay of four days, and in all three cases they were well directed.

In no case did we have to resort to a reoperation.

Only one patient presented with gastroparesis; he was put on metoclopramide and a nasogastric tube with a good evolution.

The average total hospital stay was 26 days.

Postoperative stay was 13 days.

Fourteen patients were hospitalized in the intensive care unit (44%) for an average of three days.

The post-CPD morbidity rate remains alarmingly high, varying between 27% and 35% in foreign series and between 50% and 54% in Tunisian series.

Hemorrhage is the most lethal complication, with a mortality rate of around 38%.

There are two types of hemorrhage, depending on the time of onset: early (<24 hours), which generally has a good prognosis, and late (>24 hours).

Hemorrhage may be of digestive or peritoneal origin.

Causes of haemorrhage include technical error, insufficient haemostasis or coagulopathy.

Bleeding may be secondary to loosened gastrojejunal or pancreatic-gastric anastomoses, ulcers or pseudoaneurysms.

Hemorrhage may also be secondary to injury to the gastroduodenal artery, celiac trunk, superior mesenteric artery, hepatic artery or splenic artery.

The associated factors are controversial in the literature, with all series incriminating pancreatic fistula and the presence of intra-abdominal infection or abscess.

Nevertheless, other factors may be involved: the patient's condition (male gender, advanced age, comorbidities, obesity or undernutrition), a thin diameter of the Wirsung and the duration of the operation.

Once the patient has been stabilized, an injected angioscan must precede any therapeutic decision, whether surgical or endoscopic.

PF is the most serious complication, with an incidence ranging from 1% to 36%.

It is due to disunion of the pancreatico-digestive anastomosis.

Several factors are predictive of post-CPD VT.

Some are linked to the terrain, such as obesity or recent weight loss.

They may be related to the pancreas, such as a thin diameter of the Wirsung or a soft consistency of the parenchyma.

 A pancreaticojejunal anastomosis also appears to be a predisposing factor for pancreatic fistulas.

Biliary fistula is a relatively rare complication, with an incidence of between 3% and 8%.

It is due to disunion of the hepaticojejunal anastomosis.

In the majority of cases, this is a well-tolerated complication, requiring no special treatment.

If complicated by a collection or biliary peritonitis, radiological or surgical drainage is performed.

Gastroparesis is the most frequent complication, occurring in up to 57% of cases. Treatment is based on dietary measures and the prescription of prokinetics.

Post-CPD mortality has fallen considerably over the last two decades. In foreign series, the mortality rate varies from 1% to 6%, whereas in Tunisian series it remains high, ranging from 8% to 18%.

Mortality remains closely linked to age (>75 years), the patient's condition and the occurrence of postoperative complications, especially if revision surgery is required.

It should be noted that the surgeon's experience and the selection criteria for patients undergoing CPD are determining factors in postoperative morbidity and mortality.

In conclusion, a multi-disciplinary approach is needed to combat post-CPD morbidity and mortality, with precise selection criteria.

Better patient preparation, improved surgical techniques and early management of complications can thus improve patient prognosis.

Post-CPD hemorrhage is a rare but fatal complication, and its management must involve surgeons, gastrologists, radiologists and resuscitators.

Conservative treatment should be preferred wherever possible, and greater availability of non-invasive means would reduce the risk of repeat surgery.

Close monitoring and early, systematic detection of pancreatic and biliary fistulas and gatroparesis are the best ways to prevent postoperative morbidity and mortality.

REFERENCES

1. Petermann D, Ksontini R, Halkic N, Demartines N. cephalic: indications, results and management of complications. Rev Médicale Suisse. 2008;

2. Karim SAM, Abdulla KS, Abdulkarim QH, Rahim FH. The outcomes and complications of pancreaticoduodenectomy (Whipple procedure): Cross sectional study. Int J Surg. Apr 2018;52:383-7.

3 Pappas S, Krzywda E, Mcdowell N. Nutrition and Pancreaticoduodenectomy. Nutr Clin Pract. June 2010;25(3):234-43.

4 Cristaudi A, Cerantola Y, Grass F, Hübner M, Demartines N, Schaefer M. Preoperative nutrition in visceral surgery: recommendations and reality. Rev Med Suisse. June 22, 2011;300(24):1358-61.

5 Sorensen J, Kondrup J, Prokopowicz J, Schiesser M, Krähenbühl L, Meier R, et al. EuroOOPS: An international, multicentre study to implement nutritional risk screening and evaluate clinical outcome. Clin Nutr. June 2008;27(3):340-9.

6 Barthet M, Moutardier V, Marciano S. Adenocarcinomas of the pancreas: which workup to assess resectability? Gastroentérologie Clin Biol. Feb 2007;31(2):216-21.

7. Nini E, Slim K, Belghiti J. Preoperative biliary drainage or not before cephalic duodenopancreatectomy (CPD)? Ann Chir. Dec 2003;128(10):714-5.

8. Bineshfar N, Malekpour Alamdari N, Rostami T, Mirahmadi A, Zeinalpour A. The effect of preoperative biliary drainage on postoperative complications of pancreaticoduodenectomy: a triple center retrospective study. BMC Surg. 18 Nov 2022;22(1):399.

9. Saleh MMA, N[oslash]rregaard P, J[oslash]rgensen HL, Andersen PK, Matzen P. Preoperative endoscopic stent placement before pancreaticoduodenectomy: A meta-analysis of the effect on morbidity and mortality. Gastrointest Endosc. Oct 2002;56(4):529-34.

10. Sewnath ME, Karsten TM, Prins MH, Rauws EJA, Obertop H, Gouma DJ. A Meta-analysis on the Efficacy of Preoperative Biliary Drainage for Tumors Causing Obstructive Jaundice. Ann Surg. 2002;236(1).

11. Ines K, Lamia BH, Eya C, Marie H, Samira A, Imène B, et al. Particularities of deep vein thrombosis in the elderly. Tunis Med. 2015;93.

12. Key NS, Khorana AA, Kuderer NM, Bohlke K, Lee AYY, Arcelus JI, et al. Venous Thromboembolism Prophylaxis and Treatment in Patients With Cancer: ASCO Clinical Practice Guideline Update. J Clin Oncol. Feb 10, 2020;38(5):496-520.

13. Gervaso L, Dave H, Khorana AA. Venous and Arterial Thromboembolism in Patients With Cancer. JACC CardioOncology. June 2021;3(2):173-90.

14. Gurusamy KS, Koti R, Fusai G, Davidson BR. Somatostatin analogues for pancreatic surgery. Cochrane Upper GI and Pancreatic Diseases Group, editor. Cochrane Database Syst Rev [Internet]. 30 Apr 2013 [cited 29 Mar 2023]; Available from: https://doi.wiley.com/10.1002/14651858.CD008370.pub3

15. Hüttner FJ, Fitzmaurice C, Schwarzer G, Seiler CM, Antes G, Büchler MW, et al. Pylorus-preserving pancreaticoduodenectomy (pp Whipple) versus pancreaticoduodenectomy (classic Whipple) for surgical treatment of periampullary and pancreatic carcinoma. Cochrane Upper GI and Pancreatic Diseases Group, editor. Cochrane Database Syst Rev [Internet]. 16 Feb 2016 [cited 29 Jan 2023];2016(2). Disponible sur: http://doi.wiley.com/10.1002/14651858.CD006053.pub6

16 Sastre B, Ouassi M, Pirro N, Cosentino B, Sielezneff I. Cephalic duodenopancreatectomy in the era of evidence-based medicine. Ann Chir. June 2005;130(5):295-302.

17. Christians KK, Tsai S, Tolat PP, Evans DB. Critical steps for pancreaticoduodenectomy in the setting of pancreatic adenocarcinoma: Pancreaticoduodenectomy. J Surg Oncol. 1 Jan 2013;107(1):33-8.

18. Messager M, Sabbagh C, Denost Q, Regimbeau JM, Laurent C, Rullier E, et al. What is the value of prophylactic abdominal drainage in major elective digestive surgery? J Chir Viscérale. nov 2015;152(5):316-26.

19. Wente MN, Veit JA, Bassi C, Dervenis C, Fingerhut A, Gouma DJ, et al. Postpancreatectomy hemorrhage (PPH)-An International Study Group of Pancreatic Surgery (ISGPS) definition. Surgery. July 2007;142(1):20-5.

20. Bassi C, Marchegiani G, Dervenis C, Sarr M, Abu Hilal M, Adham M, et al. The 2016 update of the International Study Group (ISGPS) definition and grading of postoperative pancreatic fistula: 11 Years After. Surgery. march 2017;161(3):584-91.

21. Russell TB, Aroori S. Procedure-specific morbidity of pancreatoduodenectomy: a systematic review of incidence and risk factors. ANZ J Surg. 2022;92(6):1347-55.

22. Herrera-Cabezón FJ, Sánchez-Acedo P, Zazpe-Ripa C, Tarifa-Castilla A, Lera-Tricas JM. Quality standards in 480 pancreatic resections: a prospective observational study. Rev Esp Enferm Dig. 2015;107.

23. Makni A. DPC technique et resultats à propos de 60 cas {thèse}. [Faculté de médecine de Tunis]: Faculté de médecine de Tunis; 2007.

24. BACCAR A. DPC morbidity and early mortality {thesis}. [Faculty of Medicine of Tunis]: Faculté de médecine de Tunis; 2016.

25. Hamdi Kbir Ghassen. DPC predictive factors mobi immediate postoperative mortality 2019 {thesis}. [Faculty of medicine of tunis]: Faculté de médecine de tunis; 2019.

26. Yang YM. Risk factors of pancreatic leakage after pancreaticoduodenectomy. World J Gastroenterol. 2005;11(16):2456.

27. Morin B, Chiche L, Salame E, Lebreton G, Rouleau V, Segol P. Carcinological results of surgical excision of cephalic glandular pancreatic cancer. Ann Chir. Nov 2006;131(9):518-23.

28. Greenblatt DY, Kelly KJ, Rajamanickam V, Wan Y, Hanson T, Rettammel R, et al. Preoperative Factors Predict Perioperative Morbidity and Mortality After Pancreaticoduodenectomy. Ann Surg Oncol. August 2011;18(8):2126-35.

29. Cameron JL, He J. Two Thousand Consecutive Pancreaticoduodenectomies. J Am Coll Surg. Apr 2015;220(4):530-6.

30. Dilek ON, Özşay O, Acar T, Gür EÖ, Çelik SC, Cengiz F, et al. Postoperative hemorrhage complications following the Whipple procedure. Turk J Surg. June 13, 2019;35(2):136-41.

31. Lee HG. Management of bleeding from pseudoaneurysms following pancreaticoduodenectomy. World J Gastroenterol. 2010;16(10):1239.

32. Wellner UF, Kulemann B, Lapshyn H, Hoeppner J, Sick O, Makowiec F, et al. Postpancreatectomy Hemorrhage-Incidence, Treatment, and Risk Factors in Over 1,000 Pancreatic Resections. J Gastrointest Surg. March 2014;18(3):464-75.

33. Feng J, Chen YL, Dong JH, Chen MY, Cai SW, Huang ZQ. Post-pancreaticoduodenectomy hemorrhage risk factors, managements and outcomes. Hepatobiliary Pancreat Dis Int. Oct 2014;13(5):513-22.

34. Uggeri F, Nespoli L, Sandini M, Andreano A, Degrate L, Romano F, et al. Analysis of risk factors for hemorrhage and related outcome after pancreatoduodenectomy in an intermediate-volume center. Updat Surg. Dec 2019;71(4):659-67.

35. Farvacque G, Guilbaud T, Loundou AD, Scemamma U, Berdah SV, Moutardier V, et al. Delayed post-pancreatectomy hemorrhage and bleeding recurrence after percutaneous endovascular treatment: risk factors from a bi-centric study of 307 consecutive patients. Langenbecks Arch Surg. Sept 2021;406(6):1893-902.

36. Gao F, Li J, Quan S, Li F, Ma D, Yao L, et al. Risk Factors and Treatment for Hemorrhage after Pancreaticoduodenectomy: A Case Series of 423 Patients. BioMed Res Int. 2016;2016:1-9.

37. Lu J, Ding H, Wu X, Liu X, Wang B, Wu Z, et al. Intra-abdominal hemorrhage following 739 consecutive pancreaticoduodenectomy: Risk factors and treatments. J Gastroenterol Hepatol. June 2019;34(6):1100-7.

38. Ball CG, Pitt HA, Kilbane ME, Dixon E, Sutherland FR, Lillemoe KD. Peri-operative blood transfusion and operative time are quality indicators for pancreatoduodenectomy. HPB. Sept 2010;12(7):465-71.

39. Boggi U, Chiaro MD, Croce C, Amorese G, Signori S, Candio GD, et al. Vascular Complications of Pancreatectomy.

40. Kamada Y, Hori T, Yamamoto H, Harada H, Yamamoto M, Yamada M, et al. Fatal arterial hemorrhage after pancreaticoduodenectomy: How do we simultaneously accomplish complete hemostasis and hepatic arterial flow? World J Hepatol. Apr 27, 2021;13(4):483-503.

41. Treckmann J, Paul A, Sotiropoulos GC, Lang H, Özcelik A, Saner F, et al. Sentinel Bleeding After Pancreaticoduodenectomy: A Disregarded Sign. J Gastrointest Surg. Feb 2008;12(2):313-8.

42. Ellison EC. Evidence-based management of hemorrhage after pancreaticoduodenectomy. Am J Surg. Jul 2007;194(1):10-2.

43. Mimatsu K, Fukino N, Kano H, Kawasaki A, Oida T. Surgical Laparotomy for Repeated Delayed Arterial Hemorrhage after Pancreaticoduodenectomy. Case Rep Gastroenterol. Feb 13, 2019;13(1):50-7.

44. Staerkle RF, Gundara JS, Hugh TJ, Maher R, Steinfort B, Samra JS. Management of recurrent bleeding after pancreatoduodenectomy: Complex post-PD bleeding. ANZ J Surg. May 2018;88(5):E435-9.

45. Mañas-Gómez MJ, Rodríguez-Revuelto R, Balsells-Valls J, Olsina-Kissler JJ, Caralt-Barba M, Pérez-Lafuente M, et al. Post-pancreaticoduodenectomy Hemorrhage. Incidence, Diagnosis, and Treatment. World J Surg. Nov 2011;35(11):2543-8.

46. Beyer L, Bonmardion R, Marciano S, Hartung O, Ramis O, Chabert L, et al. Results of Non-operative Therapy for Delayed Hemorrhage after Pancreaticoduodenectomy. J Gastrointest Surg. May 2009;13(5):922-8.

47. Hwang K, Lee JH, Hwang DW, Song KB, Kwon J, Gwon DI, et al. Clinical features and outcomes of endovascular treatment of latent pseudoaneurysmal bleeding after pancreaticoduodenectomy. ANZ J Surg [Internet]. dec 2020 [cited 3 Apr

2023];90(12). Available from: https://onlinelibrary.wiley.com/doi/10.1111/ans.16184

48. Zhou TY, Sun JH, Zhang YL, Zhou GH, Nie CH, Zhu TY, et al. Post-pancreaticoduodenectomy hemorrhage: DSA diagnosis and endovascular treatment. Oncotarget. 27 Apr 2017;8(43):73684-92.

49. Reddy JR, Saxena R, Singh RK, Pottakkat B, Prakash A, Behari A, et al. Reoperation following Pancreaticoduodenectomy. Int J Surg Oncol. 2012;2012:1-9.

50. Kawaida H, Kono H, Hosomura N, Amemiya H, Itakura J, Fujii H, et al. Surgical techniques and postoperative management to prevent postoperative pancreatic fistula after pancreatic surgery. World J Gastroenterol. 28 Jul 2019;25(28):3722-37.

51. Malgras B, Dokmak S, Aussilhou B, Pocard M, Sauvanet A. Management of postoperative pancreatic fistula after pancreaticoduodenectomy. J Visc Surg. Feb 1, 2023;160(1):39-51.

52. Bassi C, Dervenis C, Butturini G, Fingerhut A, Yeo C, Izbicki J, et al. Postoperative pancreatic fistula: An international study group (ISGPF) definition. Surgery. Jul 2005;138(1):8-13.

53. Alghamdi AA, Jawas AM, Hart RS. Use of octreotide for the prevention of pancreatic fistula after elective pancreatic surgery: a systematic review and meta-analysis.

54. Li-Ling J, Irving M. Somatostatin and octreotide in the prevention of postoperative pancreatic complications and the treatment of enterocutaneous pancreatic fistulas: a systematic review of randomized controlled trials. Br J Surg. Dec 6, 2002;88(2):190-9.

55. Ho CK, Kleeff J, Friess H, Büchler MW. Complications of pancreatic surgery. HPB. 2005;7(2):99-108.

56. Hackert T, Hinz U, Pausch T, Fesenbeck I, Strobel O, Schneider L, et al. Postoperative pancreatic fistula: We need to redefine grades B and C. Surgery. march 2016;159(3):872-7.

57. Balzano G, Pecorelli N, Piemonti L, Ariotti R, Carvello M, Nano R, et al. Relaparotomy for a pancreatic fistula after a pancreaticoduodenectomy: a comparison of different surgical strategies. HPB. jan 2014;16(1):40-5.

58. Böttger TC, Junginger T. Factors Influencing Morbidity and Mortality after Pancreaticoduodenectomy: Critical Analysis of 221 Resections. World J Surg. Feb 1999;23(2):164-72.

59. Hu BY, Wan T, Zhang WZ, Dong JH. Risk factors for postoperative pancreatic fistula: Analysis of 539 successive cases of pancreaticoduodenectomy. World J Gastroenterol. 2016;22(34):7797.

60. Callery MP, Pratt WB, Kent TS, Chaikof EL, Vollmer CM. A Prospectively Validated Clinical Risk Score Accurately Predicts Pancreatic Fistula after Pancreatoduodenectomy. J Am Coll Surg. jan 2013;216(1):1-14.

61. Lin J, Cameron J, Yeo C, Riall T, Lillemoe K. Risk factors and outcomes in postpancreaticoduodenectomy pancreaticocutaneous fistula. J Gastrointest Surg. Dec 1, 2004;8(8):951-9.

62. Gaujoux S, Cortes A, Couvelard A, Noullet S, Clavel L, Rebours V, et al. Fatty pancreas and increased body mass index are risk factors of pancreatic fistula after pancreaticoduodenectomy. Surgery. Jul 2010;148(1):15-23.

63. Fu SJ, Shen SL, Li SQ, Hu WJ, Hua YP, Kuang M, et al. Risk factors and outcomes of postoperative pancreatic fistula after pancreatico-duodenectomy: an audit of 532 consecutive cases. BMC Surg. Dec 2015;15(1):34.

64. McKay A, Mackenzie S, Sutherland FR, Bathe OF, Doig C, Dort J, et al. Meta-analysis of pancreaticojejunostomy *versus* pancreaticogastrostomy reconstruction after pancreaticoduodenectomy. Br J Surg. 17 Jul 2006;93(8):929-36.

65. El Nakeeb A, El Sorogy M, Hamed H, Said R, Elrefai M, Ezzat H, et al. Biliary leakage following pancreaticoduodenectomy: Prevalence, risk factors and management. Hepatobiliary Pancreat Dis Int. Feb 2019;18(1):67-72.

66. Wente MN, Bassi C, Dervenis C, Fingerhut A, Gouma DJ, Izbicki JR, et al. Delayed gastric emptying (DGE) after pancreatic surgery: A suggested definition by the International Study Group of Pancreatic Surgery (ISGPS). Surgery. nov 2007;142(5):761-8.

67 Petermann D, Ksontini R, Halkic N, Demartines N. Cephalic duodenopancreatectomy: indications, results and management of complications. Rev Med Suisse. June 25, 2008;163(25):1563-6.

68. Hanna MM, Gadde R, Allen CJ, Meizoso JP, Sleeman D, Livingstone AS, et al. Delayed gastric emptying after pancreaticoduodenectomy. J Surg Res. May 2016;202(2):380-8.

69. Eisenberg JD, Rosato EL, Lavu H, Yeo CJ, Winter JM. Delayed Gastric Emptying After Pancreaticoduodenectomy: an Analysis of Risk Factors and Cost. J Gastrointest Surg. Sep 1, 2015;19(9):1572-80.

70. Degisors S, Caiazzo R, Dokmak S, Truant S, Aussilhou B, Eveno C, et al. Delayed gastric emptying following distal pancreatectomy: incidence and predisposing factors. HPB. May 1, 2022;24(5):772-81.

71. Ç B, E S, O B. Risk Factors for Delayed Gastric Emptying After Pancreaticoduodenectomy. Pancreas [Internet]. Jan 5, 2022 [cited Apr 7, 2023];51(5). Available from: https://pubmed.ncbi.nlm.nih.gov/35835110/

72. Akizuki E, Kimura Y, Nobuoka T, Imamura M, Nagayama M, Sonoda T, et al. Reconsideration of Postoperative Oral Intake Tolerance After Pancreaticoduodenectomy: Prospective Consecutive Analysis of Delayed Gastric Emptying According to the ISGPS Definition and the Amount of Dietary Intake. Ann Surg. June 2009;249(6):986-94.

73. Lee YH, Hur YH, Kim HJ, Kim CY, Kim JW. Is delayed gastric emptying associated with pylorus ring preservation in patients undergoing pancreaticoduodenectomy? Asian J Surg. Jan 2021;44(1):137-42.

74. Eguchi H, Iwagami Y, Matsushita K, Tomimaru Y, Akita H, Noda T, et al. Randomized clinical trial of pancreaticogastrostomy versus pancreaticojejunostomy regarding incidence of delayed gastric emptying after pancreaticoduodenectomy. Langenbecks Arch Surg. Nov 2020;405(7):921-8.

75. Wellner UF, Sick O, Olschewski M, Adam U, Hopt UT, Keck T. Randomized Controlled Single-Center Trial Comparing Pancreatogastrostomy Versus Pancreaticojejunostomy After Partial Pancreatoduodenectomy. J Gastrointest Surg. sept 2012;16(9):1686-95.

76. Qu H, Sun GR, Zhou SQ, He QS. Clinical risk factors of delayed gastric emptying in patients after pancreaticoduodenectomy: A systematic review and meta-analysis. Eur J Surg Oncol EJSO. March 2013;39(3):213-23.

77. Lytras D, Paraskevas KI, Avgerinos C, Manes C, Touloumis Z, Paraskeva KD, et al. Therapeutic strategies for the management of delayed gastric emptying after pancreatic resection. Langenbecks Arch Surg. Jan 18, 2007;392(1):1-12.

78. Schmidt CM. Pancreaticoduodenectomy: A 20-Year Experience in 516 Patients. Arch Surg. Jul 1, 2004;139(7):718.

79. Han S liang, Zheng X feng, Shen X, Liu Z, Li J lin, Lan S hong, et al. Analysis of procedure-related complications after pancreatodoudenectomy. Indian J Surg. June 2010;72(3):194-9.

80. Simon R. Complications After Pancreaticoduodenectomy. Surg Clin North Am. 1 Oct 2021;101(5):865-74.

81. Velez-Serrano JF, Velez-Serrano D, Hernandez-Barrera V, Jimenez-Garcia R, Lopez de Andres A, Garrido PC, et al. Prediction of in-hospital mortality after pancreatic resection in pancreatic cancer patients: A boosting approach via a population-based study using health administrative data. Rocha F, editor. PLOS ONE. June 7, 2017;12(6):e0178757.

82. Wanabee DMZ Benjamin B, fistula gradeA, Ana, Ben Ali A, Mizouni A, Boudhokhan M, Nefis A, Attaoui MA, Kchaou A, Baraket O et al. CEPHALIC DUODENO PANCREATECTOMY - Monograph of the Tunisian surgical association: cephalic duodenopancreatectomy. Tunis; 2016. [Internet]. [cited 1 Apr 2023]. Available from: https://slideplayer.fr/slide/12847274/

83. Hill JS, Zhou Z, Simons JP, Ng SC, McDade TP, Whalen GF, et al. A Simple Risk Score to Predict In-Hospital Mortality After Pancreatic Resection for Cancer. Ann Surg Oncol. Jul 2010;17(7):1802-7.

84. Narayanan S, Martin AN, Turrentine FE, Bauer TW, Adams RB, Zaydfudim VM. Mortality after pancreaticoduodenectomy: assessing early and late causes of patient death. J Surg Res. Nov 2018;231:304-8.

85. Shia B, Qin L, Lin K, Fang C, Tsai L, Kao Y, et al. Age comorbidity scores as risk factors for 90-day mortality in patients with a pancreatic head adenocarcinoma receiving a pancreaticoduodenectomy: A National Population-Based Study. Cancer Med. Jan 2020;9(2):562-74.

86. Editorial Board In-hospital 30-day mortality for older patients with pancreatic cancer undergoing pancreaticoduodenectomy. J Geriatr Oncol. May 2020;11(4):IFC.

87. Nagle RT, Leiby BE, Lavu H, Rosato EL, Yeo CJ, Winter JM. Pneumonia is associated with a high risk of mortality after pancreaticoduodenectomy. Surgery. Apr 2017;161(4):959-67.

88. Kapoor VK. Complications of pancreato-duodenectomy. Rozhl V Chir Mesicnik Ceskoslovenske Chir Spolecnosti. feb 2016;95(2):53-9.

89. Halloran CM, Ghaneh P, Bosonnet L, Hartley MN, Sutton R, Neoptolemos JP. Complications of Pancreatic Cancer Resection. Dig Surg. 2002;19(2):138-46.

APPENDICES

Classically, CPP involves Whipple resection, Child reconstruction and standard lymph node curage.
CPP involves resection of the head of the pancreas, the entire duodenum, the distal part of the stomach and the bile ducts.
The lymph node curage includes resection of the retroportal lamina.

A first approach to the superior mesenteric artery (SMA) is performed for large tumors with doubt about vascular invasion.

The transverse bi-subcostal incision rather than the median approach is generally used.
The first step is exploratory to check that the tumour is respectable.

Investigation and assessment of resectability :

 The purpose of this time is to assess the technical feasibility and usefulness of an excision procedure.

- Careful palpation of the diaphragmatic cupolas, liver, peritoneum, intestine, its mesoses and the cul-de-sac of Douglas for suspicious adenopathies and grains of peritoneal carcinosis;

- Collapse of the gastrohepatic ligament at the pars flaccida, which gives access to the celiac region.

- At the submesocolic level, detachment of the first few centimetres of the jejunum enables us to grasp the superior mesenteric pedicle and look for suspicious adenopathies;

- Closer exploration of the pancreas and the lesion to assess the resectability of the pancreatic head. It requires three basic release steps:

> - complete coloepiploic detachment, freeing the right colonic angle in particular. This detachment gives access to the back cavity of the epiploons, enabling exploration of the upper side of the transverse mesocolon, the nodes of the mesenteric pedicle of the isthmus and the body of the gland;

> - Kocher manoeuvre, performed to the right flank of the aorta

- Cleavage between the anterior face of the mesentericoportal axis and the posterior face of the gland isthmus

Exeresis:

Four beats follow one another. The order in which they are performed is not constant. While most authors agree that :

- First, the head of the pancreas is freed from its biliary and hepatic arterial attachments (if only to recognize a vascular distribution anomaly that would alter the operative tactics): The gallbladder is separated from its bed anterogradely, using an electric scalpel, then the common hepatic duct is bypassed and sectioned using a cold scalpel, after ligation of the downstream side.

-Sectioning the stomach before the pancreas for reasons of exposure, the timing of jejunum section is not unanimously agreed. Sectioning it first may facilitate release of the Treitz angle and the retro-mesenteric unhooking manoeuvre.

- Pancreatic section: performed opposite the left edge of the portal vein axis, using a cold scalpel and checking for hemostasis.

- Section of the retroportal lamina: The duodenopancreatic block is grasped to expose the retroportal lamina, a dense tissue in which lymphatics, venules from the pancreatic head and posterior arterial arteries flow into the AMS.

Restoring pancreatobiliodigestive continuity: Child's approach

This is the most classic technique: the proximal jejunum drains the pancreas, the bile duct and then the stomach:
We start with a pancreatico-digestive anastomosis, in particular the pancreatico-jejunal anastomosis, followed by the hepatico-jejunal terminal-lateral anastomosis, 20 to 30 centimetres downstream of the previous one,

ending with a **gastro-jejunal anastomosis.**

And we end up **draining** it:

Systematic drainage of the peritoneal cavity after CPB is recommended(18). We usually opt for two Salem probes or two Redon drains with or without a corrugated blade.

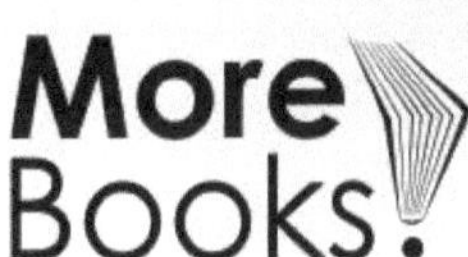

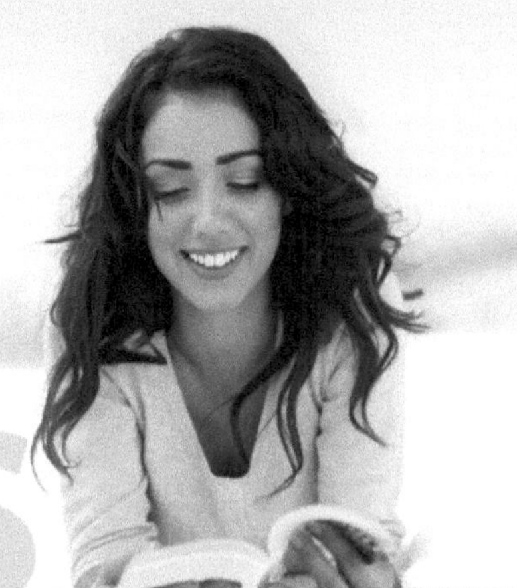

I want morebooks!

Buy your books fast and straightforward online - at one of world's fastest growing online book stores! Environmentally sound due to Print-on-Demand technologies.

Buy your books online at
www.morebooks.shop

Kaufen Sie Ihre Bücher schnell und unkompliziert online – auf einer der am schnellsten wachsenden Buchhandelsplattformen weltweit! Dank Print-On-Demand umwelt- und ressourcenschonend produzi ert.

Bücher schneller online kaufen
www.morebooks.shop

info@omniscriptum.com
www.omniscriptum.com

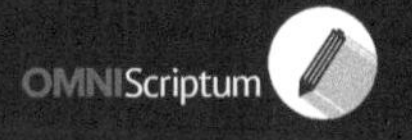

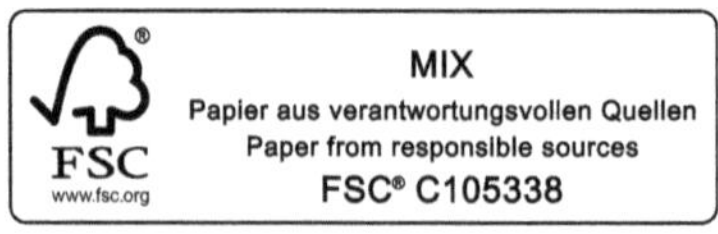

Printed by Books on Demand GmbH, Norderstedt / Germany